Ageless

Exploring Sirtuins in the Quest for Eternal Youth

A short introduction by The HealthSpan Institute

Ageless:
Exploring Sirtuins in the Quest for Eternal Youth

ISBN: 9798869707192

Printed in the United States of America

Contents

Chapter 5:
Sirtuins in Health and Disease

Chapter 6:
Activating Sirtuins–Lifestyle Choices

Chapter 7:
Pharmaceutical Pursuits–
Drugs Targeting Sirtuins

Chapter 8:
Ethics and Implications of Prolonging Human Life

Chapter 9:
Personalized Approaches to Longevity

Chapter 10:
The Future of Ageless Living

Chapter 11:
Conclusion–The Reality of Seeking Eternal Youth

Chapter 1: Introduction–The Quest for Eternal Youth

The Human Fascination with Longevity

The timeless pursuit of longevity has captivated human imagination across civilizations and epochs, reflecting an innate desire to extend life's boundaries beyond the natural confines of biological aging. This fascination, deeply rooted in the human psyche, has manifested in myths, arts, and, more recently, in scientific endeavors. The quest for eternal youth, while seemingly a modern pursuit backed by scientific rigor, is an age-old narrative that has evolved with our understanding of life and death.

Historically, the search for longevity was steeped in mysticism and legend. Ancient myths from various cultures are replete with tales of quests for magical elixirs or sacred places that promised immortality. The Epic of Gilgamesh, one of the earliest works of literature, narrates a hero's journey to find the secret of eternal life, a testament to how early human civilization was already grappling with the concept of aging and mortality. Similarly, in Chinese mythology, the pursuit of immortality was a central theme, with emperors and alchemists concocting potions in hopes of achieving eternal life.

The transition from myth to science in the quest for longevity marks a significant shift in human understanding. The Age of Enlightenment brought a more empirical approach to studying life and aging. Scientists began to view aging not as a mystical inevitability but as a biological process that could potentially be understood and controlled. This period saw the early seeds of gerontology, the study of aging, which has now blossomed into a multidisciplinary field encompassing biology, medicine, psychology, and sociology.

In the contemporary era, the fascination with longevity has taken on new dimensions with advancements in biotechnology and medicine. The mapping of the human genome and the subsequent discoveries in genetics have opened unprecedented avenues in understanding the biological mechanisms of aging. The focus has shifted from merely extending lifespan to enhancing 'healthspan' – the period of life spent in good health. Researchers are now exploring how to delay or reverse age-related decline, not just to prolong life but to improve the quality of those additional years.

The psychological underpinnings of the human obsession with longevity are as compelling as the scientific ones. Fear of death, the desire for continued experiences, and the quest for meaning and legacy are potent motivators in the pursuit of extended life. Furthermore, societal factors, such as the valorization of youth and the stigmatization of aging, fuel the desire to maintain youthfulness. In a world where aging is often associated with decline and loss, the allure of longevity promises a narrative of continued growth, productivity, and enjoyment.

However, this pursuit is not without its ethical quandaries and societal implications. The possibility of significantly extended lifespans raises questions about resource allocation, population dynamics, and intergenerational equity. There are concerns about the societal impact of a markedly increased proportion of elderly individuals and the strain it could place on social and healthcare systems. Moreover, the pursuit of longevity often highlights a disparity in access to healthcare and technology, potentially exacerbating social inequalities.

Despite these challenges, the quest for longevity continues to drive forward, now more grounded in scientific possibility than ever before. The focus on understanding and modulating aging at the molecular level, as exemplified by the study of sirtuins, signifies a new era in this quest. Sirtuins, a family of proteins, have emerged as key players in the aging process, offering potential targets for interventions to extend healthy life. The research into these molecules embodies the modern iteration of humanity's age-old dream of extending life.

In conclusion, the human fascination with longevity is a multifaceted phenomenon, deeply embedded in our cultural and psychological makeup, and now invigorated by scientific progress. From the mythical quests of ancient heroes to the cutting-edge research in molecular biology, this fascination reflects a fundamental aspect of the human condition – the desire to transcend our biological limitations. As we stand on the precipice of potentially groundbreaking discoveries in longevity, it is essential to consider the broader implications of extending life, ensuring that the quest for eternal youth benefits society as a whole, and does not exacerbate existing disparities. This journey, steeped in history and myth, now navigates uncharted scientific territories, continuing to captivate and challenge us in equal measure.

Overview of Aging Research and Sirtuins

The exploration of aging, a natural and complex process inherent to all living organisms, has long been a subject of scientific intrigue and investigation. This journey, marked by numerous discoveries and evolving theories, has more recently converged on the study of sirtuins, a group of proteins that have shown potential in influencing the aging process. Understanding the progression of aging research and the emergence of sirtuins as a focal point offers a window into the evolving landscape of longevity studies.

The scientific investigation of aging began with the quest to understand the fundamental causes of aging at a cellular and molecular level. Early research centered on theories like the wear and tear hypothesis, which likened aging to the gradual deterioration of living cells and tissues, similar to the aging of inanimate objects. However, this simplistic view was soon supplanted by more sophisticated theories as the field of biology advanced.

One significant milestone in aging research was the free radical theory of aging, proposed by Denham Harman in the 1950s. This theory suggested that aging results from the accumulation of damage caused by free radicals–unstable molecules that can cause significant damage to cellular components. This theory spurred a vast amount of research into antioxidants as potential anti-aging agents.

However, the landscape of aging research experienced a paradigm shift with the advent of genetic research. The discovery that certain genetic mutations could extend the lifespan of model organisms like the nematode C. elegans suggested that aging might be regulated by specific genetic pathways. This revelation steered the scientific community towards a genetic approach to understanding aging.

It is within this genetic context that sirtuins emerged as critical players. Sirtuins, first discovered in the early 1990s, are a family of proteins that play diverse roles in cellular regulation, including DNA repair, metabolism, and inflammation. These proteins, particularly the sirtuin known as SIRT1, gained prominence due to their role in regulating the aging process.

The link between sirtuins and aging was first observed in yeast, where increasing the activity of a sirtuin gene extended the organism's lifespan. This finding was groundbreaking, suggesting that the manipulation of certain genes could influence longevity. Further research in other model organisms, including flies and mice, corroborated the potential of sirtuins in modulating aging.

Sirtuins function as NAD+-dependent deacetylases, meaning they remove acetyl groups from proteins in a process that requires NAD+, a coenzyme found in all living cells. This activity is crucial in cellular stress responses and energy metabolism, both of which are integral to the aging process. Additionally, sirtuins have been implicated in the regulation of circadian rhythms and inflammatory processes, both known to play roles in aging and age-related diseases.

The connection between sirtuins and caloric restriction, a well-known intervention that extends lifespan in various organisms, further underscores their significance in aging research. Caloric restriction has been shown to activate sirtuins, suggesting that these proteins might mediate some of the anti-aging effects of reduced calorie intake.

Despite the excitement surrounding sirtuins, the field has faced challenges and controversies. Initial claims about the life-extending properties of resveratrol, a compound thought to activate SIRT1, were met with skepticism and conflicting results in subsequent studies. These challenges highlight the complexities of aging research and the need for cautious interpretation of data.

The study of sirtuins has also expanded to explore their role in age-related diseases, such as neurodegenerative disorders, cardiovascular diseases, and diabetes. This line of research holds promise not only for extending lifespan but also for improving healthspan–the period of life spent in good health.

In conclusion, the journey of aging research from its early theories to the current focus on sirtuins illustrates the evolving understanding of this complex biological process. Sirtuins, with their multifaceted roles in cellular function and potential to influence longevity, represent a significant frontier in the quest to decipher the mysteries of aging. As researchers continue to unravel the intricate mechanisms by which sirtuins affect the aging process, the hope is not only to extend human lifespan but also to enhance the quality of life in the later years. This endeavor, rooted in scientific curiosity and the age-old human desire to conquer the bounds of aging, continues to be a compelling chapter in the ongoing narrative of aging research.

Chapter 2: Unraveling the Mystery of Sirtuins

What Are Sirtuins?

Sirtuins, a family of proteins that have garnered significant attention in the field of aging research, represent a fascinating aspect of cellular biology with implications that extend far beyond the boundaries of longevity science. These proteins, known for their regulatory roles in various cellular processes, have become a cornerstone in the study of aging and metabolic regulation. This essay delves into the nature of sirtuins, exploring their functions, mechanisms of action, and the potential they hold in influencing human health and aging.

Sirtuins were initially identified in yeast as a type of protein involved in gene silencing, a process by which cells regulate the expression of certain genes. This discovery marked the beginning of a journey into understanding the diverse functions of these proteins. In humans, there are seven known sirtuins, named SIRT1 to SIRT7, each with unique functions and localizations within the cell. These proteins are present in various cellular compartments, including the nucleus, cytoplasm, and mitochondria, reflecting their diverse roles in cellular physiology.

The primary function of sirtuins is to act as NAD+-dependent deacetylases. Acetylation, the addition of an acetyl group to a molecule, is a common type of post-translational modification that can alter the function of proteins. Sirtuins remove these acetyl groups in a process that depends on NAD+, a coenzyme involved in cellular energy metabolism. This link between sirtuins and cellular energy status is key to understanding their role in aging and metabolism.

One of the most well-studied sirtuins is SIRT1, which is known for its involvement in DNA repair, gene expression regulation, and inflammatory responses. SIRT1 has been shown to protect cells from oxidative stress and DNA damage, processes that are central to the aging phenomenon. It also regulates the activity of several transcription factors and co-regulators, influencing the expression of genes involved in metabolism, stress responses, and cell survival.

SIRT3, predominantly located in the mitochondria – the cell's powerhouse – plays a vital role in regulating mitochondrial function and energy production. By deacetylating and activating various enzymes in the mitochondria, SIRT3 contributes to efficient energy production and protection against oxidative stress, a significant factor in the aging process.

The functions of sirtuins extend beyond their roles in aging and metabolism. For instance, SIRT6 is involved in maintaining genomic stability and DNA repair, while SIRT7 has been implicated in the regulation of ribosomal RNA transcription, a critical process for protein synthesis in cells.

Research on sirtuins has also highlighted their involvement in various age-related diseases. Dysregulation of sirtuin activity has been linked to neurodegenerative disorders, cardiovascular diseases, and metabolic syndromes. This connection suggests that modulation of sirtuin activity could be a potential therapeutic strategy for these conditions.

The interest in sirtuins has led to the exploration of ways to modulate their activity. Compounds such as resveratrol, a polyphenol found in red wine, have been studied for their potential to activate sirtuins, particularly SIRT1. While initial studies were promising, suggesting that resveratrol could mimic the effects of caloric restriction and extend lifespan, later research has yielded mixed results, emphasizing the complexity of sirtuin biology.

Despite the challenges, the study of sirtuins continues to be a dynamic and evolving field. Scientists are exploring novel sirtuin-activating compounds, delving into the intricate mechanisms by which these proteins influence aging and disease processes. This research holds the promise of uncovering new therapeutic avenues for age-related diseases and possibly extending healthspan.

In conclusion, sirtuins represent a pivotal element in the complex machinery of cellular biology. Their diverse roles in regulating metabolism, stress responses, DNA repair, and gene expression position them at the crossroads of aging and disease. As research continues to unravel the multifaceted nature of these proteins, the potential to leverage their functions for improving human health and longevity remains an exciting and promising prospect. The exploration of sirtuins is not just a scientific endeavor; it's a journey into understanding the fundamental processes that govern life and aging, offering a glimpse into the possibilities of extending healthy human life.

Historical Discovery and Evolution of Sirtuin Research

The journey of sirtuin research, a field integral to our understanding of aging and longevity, is a fascinating tale of scientific discovery and evolution. Spanning several decades, this narrative is a testament to how incremental advances in science can lead to significant breakthroughs in our understanding of complex biological processes. The story of sirtuins is not just a chronicle of molecular biology but also a reflection of the changing perspectives on aging and longevity.

The origin of sirtuin research can be traced back to the 1970s, although the significance of these proteins was not understood until much later. Initially, sirtuins were discovered in the context of gene regulation in yeast. Leonard Guarente and colleagues at the Massachusetts Institute of Technology were among the first to explore the role of these proteins, identifying them as regulators of gene silencing in yeast. This discovery was a pivotal moment, laying the groundwork for understanding the broader implications of sirtuins in cellular biology.

However, the true potential of sirtuins began to emerge in the late 1990s and early 2000s, when researchers started to unravel their roles beyond yeast and gene silencing. This period marked a shift from a focus on basic yeast biology to a broader interest in sirtuins as regulators of aging and longevity. The landmark study that propelled sirtuins into the limelight was the discovery of their role in mediating the effects of caloric restriction on lifespan extension in model organisms. This finding was groundbreaking, as it linked sirtuins directly to the aging process and suggested a potential mechanism for the well-documented lifespan-extending effects of caloric restriction.

The early 2000s witnessed a surge in sirtuin research, with scientists exploring the functions of different sirtuins in various organisms, including mammals. The discovery of seven sirtuins in humans (SIRT1-7), each with distinct functions and localizations in the cell, revealed the complexity of these proteins. Research during this period began to highlight the diverse roles of sirtuins in DNA repair, metabolism, stress resistance, and inflammation, all of which are processes implicated in aging.

One of the most significant developments in sirtuin research was the discovery of their enzymatic activity. Sirtuins were found to be NAD+-dependent deacetylases, linking their activity to the cell's metabolic state. This finding was crucial as it provided a molecular explanation for how sirtuins could sense and respond to changes in cellular energy levels, a key aspect of their role in aging and metabolism.

The mid-2000s to the 2010s saw a rapid expansion in sirtuin research, with numerous studies exploring their molecular mechanisms and potential therapeutic applications. The hype around sirtuins peaked with the discovery of small molecules like resveratrol, which were thought to activate SIRT1 and mimic the effects of caloric restriction. This period was marked by a mix of excitement and controversy, as some early findings were later challenged or nuanced by further research.

Despite the controversies, the interest in sirtuins persisted, driven by the potential implications for human health and longevity. Researchers continued to explore the roles of different sirtuins in various age-related diseases, including neurodegenerative disorders, cardiovascular diseases, and metabolic syndromes. This line of research highlighted the potential of targeting sirtuins for therapeutic purposes.

The evolution of sirtuin research also reflects the broader changes in the field of aging research. Initially considered a niche area within biology, the study of aging has now become a major interdisciplinary field, with sirtuins at its core. The growing interest in understanding and potentially manipulating the aging process for health benefits has positioned sirtuins as a critical area of investigation.

In conclusion, the historical discovery and evolution of sirtuin research is a narrative of scientific progress, marked by both excitement and skepticism. From their initial identification in yeast to their recognition as key regulators of aging and metabolism in humans, sirtuins have become central to our understanding of the biological underpinnings of aging. As research continues to uncover the intricate details of sirtuin biology, the potential to harness these proteins for improving human health and longevity remains an exciting and evolving area of scientific inquiry. The story of sirtuins is far from complete, and future research promises to add new chapters to this fascinating saga.

Chapter 3: Sirtuins–At the Heart of Cellular Function

Understanding the Biology of Sirtuins

Sirtuins, a captivating group of proteins, play a pivotal role in the intricate network of cellular functions. Their discovery and subsequent research have unveiled a wealth of information about their multifaceted roles in various biological processes. Understanding the biology of sirtuins is crucial for comprehending their impact on aging, metabolism, and disease. This essay delves into the complex world of sirtuins, elucidating their structure, functions, and mechanisms of action, thereby highlighting their significance in cellular biology.

At the heart of sirtuin biology is their unique structure and enzymatic activity. Sirtuins are characterized by a conserved sirtuin core domain, which is responsible for their enzymatic functions. The core domain contains a series of folds that bind to nicotinamide adenine dinucleotide (NAD+), a critical coenzyme in cellular metabolism. This dependency on NAD+ links sirtuins' activity to the metabolic state of the cell, making them sensitive to changes in cellular energy levels.

The primary function of sirtuins as NAD+-dependent deacetylases involves the removal of acetyl groups from specific protein substrates. This deacetylation process is crucial for regulating various cellular functions. Acetylation, the addition of acetyl groups to lysine residues on proteins, is a common post-translational modification that can affect protein stability, localization, and activity. By removing these acetyl groups, sirtuins can modulate the function of numerous proteins, impacting processes such as gene expression, DNA repair, and metabolic regulation.

SIRT1, the most extensively studied sirtuin, exemplifies the diverse roles these proteins play. Located primarily in the nucleus, SIRT1 influences cellular health by regulating the activity of transcription factors and co-regulators. It plays a key role in stress responses, particularly in DNA repair and chromatin remodeling. SIRT1's ability to sense the cell's nutritional status and adapt gene expression accordingly positions it as a crucial mediator of cellular homeostasis.

SIRT3, SIRT4, and SIRT5, predominantly mitochondrial sirtuins, are central to maintaining mitochondrial integrity and function. Mitochondria are not only the powerhouse of the cell but also pivotal in apoptosis, calcium signaling, and reactive oxygen species (ROS) production. SIRT3, for instance, deacetylates and activates various enzymes involved in the Krebs cycle and electron transport chain, optimizing mitochondrial energy production and reducing oxidative stress. This activity is crucial for preventing mitochondrial dysfunction, a hallmark of aging and many age-related diseases.

The functions of sirtuins also extend to the regulation of lipid metabolism and insulin sensitivity, as seen with SIRT1 and SIRT6. Their involvement in lipid metabolism is particularly significant given the rising prevalence of metabolic disorders such as obesity and diabetes. By modulating the activity of factors involved in fatty acid oxidation and insulin secretion, sirtuins can influence the body's metabolic balance, offering potential therapeutic targets for metabolic diseases.

Another intriguing aspect of sirtuin biology is their role in inflammation and stress resistance. Sirtuins regulate the activity of NF-κB, a key transcription factor in the inflammatory response. By modulating NF-κB signaling, sirtuins can influence the immune response and cellular stress pathways, providing a link between metabolism, inflammation, and aging.

The study of sirtuins has also expanded to include their involvement in circadian rhythms. Circadian rhythms, the physiological processes that follow a roughly 24-hour cycle, are fundamental to maintaining cellular and systemic homeostasis. Sirtuins, particularly SIRT1, have been shown to interact with core components of the circadian clock, suggesting a role in synchronizing metabolic processes with the body's internal clock.

Despite the significant progress in understanding sirtuin biology, many questions remain. The complexity of their regulatory networks, their interaction with other cellular pathways, and the context-dependent nature of their activity present ongoing challenges. Moreover, the potential therapeutic manipulation of sirtuins in human health and disease requires a deeper understanding of their functions and regulatory mechanisms.

In conclusion, the biology of sirtuins is a testament to the complexity and interconnectivity of cellular processes. From regulating gene expression and DNA repair to modulating metabolism and inflammation, sirtuins are integral players in the maintenance of cellular health and function. As research continues to unravel the intricate details of sirtuin biology, the potential for harnessing these proteins in therapeutic interventions for aging and age-related diseases becomes increasingly apparent. The study of sirtuins not only offers insights into the fundamental processes of life but also opens up new avenues for improving human health and longevity.

Types of Sirtuins and Their Roles in the Cell

Sirtuins, a family of proteins integral to cellular function, have emerged as key regulators in a myriad of biological processes. These proteins, known for their NAD+-dependent deacetylase activity, play diverse roles in the cell, impacting aging, metabolism, DNA repair, and stress resistance. In humans, seven distinct sirtuins (SIRT1-7) have been identified, each possessing unique functions and localizations within the cell. This essay explores the varied types of sirtuins and their specific roles, underscoring their significance in cellular biology.

SIRT1: The Multifaceted Regulator

SIRT1, perhaps the most well-known sirtuin, is predominantly located in the nucleus. It modulates various aspects of cellular physiology, including gene expression, DNA repair, and apoptosis. SIRT1 regulates the activity of several transcription factors and co-regulators, such as p53, NF-κB, and FOXO, thereby influencing cellular stress responses, inflammation, and metabolism. Its role in caloric restriction-mediated lifespan extension has garnered significant attention, positioning SIRT1 as a central player in aging research.

SIRT2: The Cytoplasmic Guardian

SIRT2, primarily found in the cytoplasm, is involved in the regulation of the cell cycle and cytoskeletal organization. It deacetylates α-tubulin, influencing microtubule dynamics, which is crucial for cell division and intracellular transport. SIRT2 also plays a role in metabolic regulation, particularly in the context of lipid metabolism and insulin signaling, making it a protein of interest in the study of metabolic diseases.

SIRT3: The Mitochondrial Protector

SIRT3 is a mitochondrial sirtuin that plays a vital role in regulating mitochondrial metabolism and oxidative stress. It deacetylates and activates several enzymes involved in the Krebs cycle, fatty acid oxidation, and the electron transport chain. By optimizing mitochondrial function, SIRT3 contributes to cellular energy efficiency and protection against oxidative damage, which is pivotal in aging and age-related disorders.

SIRT4: The Metabolic Regulator

Also located in the mitochondria, SIRT4 has a unique role compared to other sirtuins. It lacks robust deacetylase activity but possesses ADP-ribosyltransferase activity. SIRT4 regulates insulin secretion and amino acid metabolism by modulating enzymes involved in the urea cycle and fatty acid metabolism. Its role in cellular metabolism and energy homeostasis makes SIRT4 an interesting target for metabolic and aging research.

SIRT5: The Versatile Modifier

SIRT5, another mitochondrial sirtuin, is unique in its enzymatic activity. It primarily functions as a demalonylase, desuccinylase, and deglutarylase, removing modifications other than acetyl groups. SIRT5 regulates various aspects of mitochondrial metabolism, including ammonia detoxification and oxidative stress response. Its distinct enzymatic capabilities broaden the scope of sirtuin-mediated post-translational modifications, highlighting the complexity of cellular regulation.

SIRT6: The Genome Stabilizer

SIRT6, predominantly found in the nucleus, is essential for maintaining genomic stability. It is involved in DNA repair, telomere maintenance, and chromatin remodeling. SIRT6 regulates the activity of NF-κB, influencing inflammation and aging. Additionally, it modulates glucose metabolism by influencing the expression of genes involved in glycolysis and insulin signaling, underscoring its role in metabolic health.

SIRT7: The Transcriptional Regulator

SIRT7 is primarily localized in the nucleolus and is involved in regulating RNA polymerase I-mediated transcription, essential for ribosomal RNA synthesis. It plays a role in maintaining cellular homeostasis under stress conditions and has been implicated in cardiac function and lipid metabolism. SIRT7's specific role in the nucleolus highlights the diverse cellular localizations and functions of sirtuins.

Each sirtuin, with its distinct localization and functional repertoire, contributes to the intricate network of cellular regulation. Their roles in metabolism, stress response, DNA repair, and cell cycle regulation are crucial for maintaining cellular homeostasis and responding to environmental changes. The diverse enzymatic activities of sirtuins, extending beyond deacetylation to include ADP-ribosylation, demalonylation, desuccinylation, and deglutarylation, reflect the complexity of post-translational modifications in cellular regulation.

The study of sirtuins has evolved from a focus on their roles in lifespan extension to a broader exploration of their impact on cellular and organismal health. Their involvement in age-related diseases, such as neurodegeneration, cardiovascular disorders, and metabolic syndromes, makes them potential targets for therapeutic intervention. The ongoing research into sirtuins continues to unravel their multifaceted roles, offering insights into the molecular mechanisms underpinning health

Chapter 4: Sirtuins and the Aging Process

How Sirtuins Influence Aging

The exploration of how sirtuins influence aging represents a crucial aspect of modern biogerontology. These proteins, belonging to a class known for their NAD+-dependent deacetylase activity, are deeply intertwined with various cellular processes that are central to the aging phenomenon. The relationship between sirtuins and aging is a multifaceted one, encompassing aspects of gene expression, DNA repair, metabolic regulation, and stress resistance. This essay delves into the intricate mechanisms by which sirtuins exert their influence on aging, highlighting the profound impact these proteins have on the aging process.

The connection between sirtuins and aging first came into the spotlight with the discovery of their role in caloric restriction (CR), a well-documented method for extending lifespan in various organisms. CR has been shown to increase the activity of sirtuins, particularly SIRT1, suggesting that these proteins may mediate some of the beneficial effects of CR on lifespan. Sirtuins, by sensing changes in the cellular energy status via NAD+ levels, can modulate cellular functions in response to metabolic changes. This ability to respond to metabolic cues is central to their role in the aging process.

At the genetic level, sirtuins influence aging through their impact on gene expression. SIRT1, for instance, modulates the activity of several transcription factors, including those involved in stress responses and metabolic regulation. By deacetylating histones and transcription factors, SIRT1 can alter the expression of genes associated with longevity and stress resistance. This regulation of gene expression is key to maintaining cellular homeostasis and adapting to environmental stressors, both of which are critical in the aging process.

Another significant aspect of sirtuins' influence on aging is their role in DNA repair and genomic stability. Aging is associated with the accumulation of DNA damage, and the ability to efficiently repair this damage is essential for longevity. Sirtuins, particularly SIRT6, are involved in DNA repair mechanisms. SIRT6, for example, has been shown to promote DNA double-strand break repair and maintain telomere integrity, both of which are crucial for preventing the genomic instability that characterizes aging cells.

Sirtuins also play a vital role in mitochondrial function, which is closely linked to the aging process. Mitochondrial dysfunction is a hallmark of aging, characterized by decreased energy production and increased oxidative stress. SIRT3, a mitochondrial sirtuin, enhances the efficiency of oxidative phosphorylation and reduces the production of reactive oxygen species (ROS), thereby protecting cells from oxidative damage. By maintaining mitochondrial health, sirtuins like SIRT3 contribute to cellular longevity and resistance to age-related decline.

The regulation of metabolism is another pathway through which sirtuins influence aging. Sirtuins modulate various metabolic processes, including fat and glucose metabolism, which are often dysregulated with age. By influencing pathways such as insulin signaling and fatty acid oxidation, sirtuins can enhance metabolic efficiency and protect against metabolic diseases, which are major contributors to age-related morbidity.

In addition to these direct effects on cellular processes, sirtuins also exert indirect effects on aging through their influence on inflammation and stress resistance. Chronic, low-grade inflammation is a characteristic feature of aging, known as "inflammaging." Sirtuins, particularly SIRT1 and SIRT6, have anti-inflammatory properties, modulating the activity of NF-κB and other inflammatory pathways. By mitigating inflammatory responses, sirtuins can counteract one of the key drivers of aging and age-related diseases.

The complex interplay between sirtuins and the aging process is not just of academic interest but has significant implications for therapeutic interventions in aging and age-related diseases. Understanding how sirtuins modulate the aging process opens the possibility of manipulating these pathways to promote healthy aging and longevity. For instance, pharmacological activators of sirtuins, such as resveratrol and other small molecules, have been explored as potential anti-aging interventions.

In conclusion, sirtuins play a multifaceted and influential role in the aging process. Their ability to modulate gene expression, DNA repair, metabolism, and stress responses positions them as central regulators of cellular aging. The ongoing research into sirtuins continues to unravel the complex mechanisms by which these proteins influence aging, offering the potential for novel interventions in aging and age-related diseases. As our understanding of sirtuins deepens, so does our ability to influence the aging process, potentially paving the way for more effective strategies to promote health and longevity.

Key Studies Linking Sirtuins to Longevity

The exploration of sirtuins and their connection to longevity is a dynamic and rapidly evolving field within aging research. Several key studies have been instrumental in establishing this link, providing insights into the molecular mechanisms underlying the aging process and potential interventions for extending healthy lifespan. These studies span various models, from yeast to mammals, and have significantly advanced our understanding of how sirtuins influence longevity.

Early Discoveries in Yeast and Worms

The foundational studies linking sirtuins to longevity began with research on yeast, specifically the discovery of the SIR2 gene. Leonard Guarente and colleagues at the Massachusetts Institute of Technology first noted that increased expression of SIR2 extended the replicative lifespan of yeast. This was a pivotal finding, as it suggested a genetic basis for lifespan extension and introduced the concept that aging might be modifiable at the molecular level.

Following these yeast studies, researchers turned their attention to Caenorhabditis elegans, a nematode worm commonly used in aging research. In a landmark study, researchers found that overexpression of sir-2.1, the worm equivalent of the SIR2 gene, extended the lifespan of these organisms. This study was critical in demonstrating that the role of sirtuins in longevity was not limited to yeast but was also relevant in more complex organisms.

Insights from Drosophila and Mammalian Models

The role of sirtuins in aging was further elucidated through studies in Drosophila melanogaster, the fruit fly. Researchers observed that increasing the activity of the fly's version of the SIR2 gene also led to lifespan extension. These findings in Drosophila reinforced the notion that the longevity-promoting effects of sirtuins were conserved across species.

In mammalian models, particularly mice, the investigation of sirtuins took a more complex turn, given the presence of seven different sirtuins (SIRT1-7) with distinct functions. Mice studies have been instrumental in understanding the diverse roles of these sirtuins in aging and longevity. For example, mice overexpressing SIRT1 exhibited improved healthspan, characterized by a reduction in age-related pathologies. Similarly, mice with enhanced SIRT6 expression showed increased lifespan and resistance to age-related diseases.

The Caloric Restriction Connection

A key aspect of sirtuin research in the context of longevity is their connection to caloric restriction (CR), a well-established method for extending lifespan in various species. Studies have shown that CR increases the activity of sirtuins, particularly SIRT1, suggesting that these proteins mediate some of the beneficial effects of CR on lifespan. This link has provided a mechanistic understanding of how CR influences aging and has spurred research into mimetics that can activate sirtuins to mimic the effects of CR.

Human Studies and Clinical Implications

While most of the foundational research on sirtuins and longevity has been conducted in model organisms, recent studies have begun to explore their relevance in humans. Epidemiological studies have associated variants in sirtuin genes with longevity in human populations. Additionally, research into age-related diseases, such as Alzheimer's disease and cardiovascular disease, has highlighted the potential role of sirtuins in modulating disease processes and influencing lifespan.

Controversies and Evolving Perspectives

The journey of sirtuin research has not been without controversy. Initial studies suggesting that compounds like resveratrol, a sirtuin activator, could extend lifespan in mammals were met with excitement, but subsequent research provided mixed results. These controversies have highlighted the complexities of translating findings from model organisms to humans and the need for a nuanced understanding of sirtuin biology.

Future Directions

The ongoing research into sirtuins and longevity continues to evolve, with a focus on understanding the precise mechanisms by which these proteins influence aging and identifying potential therapeutic targets. The development of specific sirtuin activators and inhibitors, and their testing in clinical trials, represents a promising area of research with the potential to translate these findings into interventions for age-related diseases and lifespan extension.

In conclusion, the body of research linking sirtuins to longevity is extensive and continues to grow. From initial discoveries in yeast to complex studies in mammals, these investigations have significantly advanced our understanding of the aging process. The diverse roles of sirtuins in cellular function, their connection to caloric restriction, and their potential implications for human health and aging make them a focal point in the quest to understand and modulate the aging process. As research advances, it holds the promise of uncovering new strategies for promoting health and longevity, potentially transforming our approach to aging and age-related diseases.

Chapter 5: Sirtuins in Health and Disease

Sirtuins in Preventing Age-Related Diseases

Sirtuins, a family of proteins renowned for their role in aging, have garnered significant attention for their potential in preventing age-related diseases. The increasing understanding of how sirtuins function at the molecular level has revealed their profound impact on various cellular processes associated with aging and age-related pathologies. This essay explores the critical roles of sirtuins in preventing and potentially treating a range of age-related diseases, shedding light on their therapeutic potential.

Sirtuins and Neurodegenerative Diseases

One of the most promising areas of sirtuin research is their role in neurodegenerative diseases such as Alzheimer's and Parkinson's disease. These conditions are characterized by the progressive loss of neuronal function and are closely linked to aging. Sirtuins, particularly SIRT1 and SIRT3, have been shown to have neuroprotective properties. They are involved in regulating oxidative stress, mitochondrial function, and inflammation, all of which are key factors in the pathogenesis of neurodegenerative diseases. For instance, SIRT1 activation has been found to enhance the clearance of amyloid-beta plaques, a hallmark of Alzheimer's disease. Additionally, sirtuins regulate the activity of factors involved in neuronal plasticity and survival, suggesting their potential in mitigating the progression of neurodegenerative conditions.

Impact on Cardiovascular Health

Cardiovascular diseases, the leading cause of mortality globally, are intimately linked with aging. Sirtuins, especially SIRT1 and SIRT6, have been implicated in promoting cardiovascular health. They modulate various aspects of cardiovascular function, including endothelial function, cholesterol homeostasis, and response to oxidative stress. For example, SIRT1 activation has been associated with improved endothelial function and reduced atherosclerosis, while SIRT6 has been found to protect against cardiac hypertrophy and heart failure. By targeting the underlying mechanisms of cardiovascular aging, sirtuins hold promise for preventing and managing age-related cardiovascular diseases.

Sirtuins in Metabolic Syndrome and Diabetes

Metabolic syndrome, a cluster of conditions including obesity, insulin resistance, and dyslipidemia, is a major risk factor for various age-related diseases, including type 2 diabetes. Sirtuins, particularly SIRT1, play a crucial role in regulating metabolic homeostasis. They are involved in glucose and lipid metabolism, influencing insulin sensitivity and adipogenesis. Activation of sirtuins has been shown to improve metabolic profiles in animal models, suggesting their potential in preventing and treating metabolic disorders. Furthermore, sirtuins modulate inflammatory pathways associated with obesity and metabolic syndrome, providing a multi-faceted approach to managing these conditions.

Role in Cancer Prevention

The relationship between sirtuins and cancer is complex, given that they can have both tumor-promoting and tumor-suppressing functions. However, in the context of age-related cancer prevention, sirtuins play a significant role. They are involved in DNA repair, chromatin remodeling, and the regulation of cellular senescence and apoptosis, all of which are critical in preventing the onset and progression of cancer. For example, SIRT6 has been shown to maintain genomic stability and suppress tumorigenesis. The modulation of sirtuins could thus represent a novel strategy in cancer prevention, particularly in the context of aging.

Mitigating Inflammation and Immune Aging

Chronic inflammation is a characteristic feature of aging and is implicated in the pathogenesis of many age-related diseases. Sirtuins, especially SIRT1 and SIRT6, have anti-inflammatory properties, modulating key inflammatory pathways and cytokine production. Through their regulatory effects on NF-κB and other inflammatory mediators, sirtuins can mitigate chronic inflammation, thereby potentially preventing a range of age-related diseases, including autoimmune and neurodegenerative disorders.

Future Perspectives and Challenges

The potential of sirtuins in preventing age-related diseases is vast, yet there are challenges and considerations in translating these findings into clinical applications. The complexity of sirtuin biology, with their diverse and sometimes contradictory roles, requires a nuanced understanding of their functions in different contexts. Additionally, the development of specific sirtuin modulators for therapeutic use necessitates careful consideration of potential side effects and long-term impacts.

Conclusion

In conclusion, sirtuins represent a significant frontier in the fight against age-related diseases. Their roles in regulating key processes associated with aging, from metabolic regulation to DNA repair and inflammation, position them as critical players in maintaining health during aging. The ongoing research into sirtuins and their modulation offers hope for novel interventions in a range of age-related conditions, potentially transforming our approach to aging and age-related disease management. As our understanding of these complex proteins deepens, so does the possibility of harnessing their power to improve health and longevity.

Role in Metabolism, DNA Repair, and Neuroprotection

Sirtuins, a class of proteins deeply embedded in the regulatory networks of the cell, have gained prominence for their roles in metabolism, DNA repair, and neuroprotection. These functions are not only crucial for maintaining cellular health but also play a pivotal role in preventing and potentially treating age-related diseases. The study of sirtuins in these areas has unveiled a complex but fascinating picture of how these proteins influence health and disease. This essay delves into the multifaceted roles of sirtuins in metabolism, DNA repair, and neuroprotection, highlighting their significance in cellular function and potential therapeutic applications.

Sirtuins in Metabolic Regulation

Metabolism is a fundamental cellular process involving the conversion of nutrients into energy and building blocks necessary for cell growth, reproduction, and maintenance. Sirtuins play a key role in regulating metabolism, responding to changes in nutrient availability and energy demands. SIRT1, in particular, is a critical regulator of glucose and lipid metabolism. It influences insulin secretion and sensitivity, key factors in metabolic disorders like diabetes. SIRT1 also regulates the activity of PGC-1α, a coactivator involved in mitochondrial biogenesis and function, underscoring its role in energy homeostasis.

Sirtuins also modulate lipid metabolism, affecting processes like fatty acid oxidation and adipogenesis. SIRT6, for example, has been shown to suppress fat accumulation and improve lipid profiles, indicating its potential role in combating obesity and related metabolic conditions. By influencing these metabolic pathways, sirtuins not only impact energy balance but also affect the overall metabolic health of the organism, making them key targets for intervention in metabolic diseases.

DNA Repair and Genomic Stability

DNA repair is a vital cellular defense mechanism against genomic instability, a major contributor to aging and cancer. Sirtuins, particularly SIRT6 and SIRT1, play significant roles in maintaining genomic stability. SIRT6 has been shown to be involved in base excision repair, a pathway critical for repairing DNA damage caused by oxidative stress. It also helps in maintaining the integrity of telomeres, the protective ends of chromosomes, which are known to shorten with age.

SIRT1, on the other hand, participates in various DNA repair processes, including double-strand break repair. It modulates the activity of proteins involved in the DNA damage response, such as PARP1 and NBS1. By ensuring effective DNA repair and maintaining genomic stability, sirtuins protect cells from the accumulative damage that characterizes aging and contributes to cancer development.

Neuroprotection and Brain Health

The role of sirtuins in neuroprotection is a rapidly growing area of interest, particularly in the context of neurodegenerative diseases. Sirtuins, especially SIRT1 and SIRT3, exhibit neuroprotective properties by modulating oxidative stress, mitochondrial function, and inflammatory responses in the brain. SIRT1 has been shown to protect neurons from degeneration in models of Alzheimer's disease and Huntington's disease. It achieves this by influencing pathways involved in amyloid-beta clearance, tau phosphorylation, and neuronal survival.

SIRT3, primarily located in mitochondria, is crucial for maintaining mitochondrial function in neurons. It regulates the production of reactive oxygen species and enhances the antioxidant capacity of cells, protecting neurons from oxidative damage, a common feature in neurodegenerative disorders.

Furthermore, sirtuins are involved in modulating synaptic plasticity and cognitive functions. They influence the expression of genes involved in learning and memory, suggesting their potential role in combating cognitive decline associated with aging and neurodegenerative diseases.

Therapeutic Potential and Challenges

The diverse roles of sirtuins in metabolism, DNA repair, and neuroprotection present them as attractive targets for therapeutic intervention in a range of diseases. Developing sirtuin activators or inhibitors could offer new avenues for treating metabolic disorders, neurodegenerative diseases, and conditions related to genomic instability such as cancer.

However, translating these findings into clinical applications poses significant challenges. The pleiotropic nature of sirtuins means that modulating their activity could have wide-ranging effects, some of which might be detrimental. Additionally, the efficacy and safety of sirtuin-targeted therapies need thorough evaluation in clinical settings.

Conclusion

In conclusion, sirtuins play critical roles in regulating metabolism, ensuring DNA repair, and providing neuroprotection. These functions are central to maintaining cellular health and preventing a range of age-related diseases. The ongoing research into sirtuins continues to reveal their complex roles in cellular physiology and their potential as targets for therapeutic intervention. As our understanding of these versatile proteins deepens, so does the possibility of harnessing their power to improve human health and treat diseases. The exploration of sirtuins stands at the forefront of aging research, offering hope for new strategies to combat the challenges of aging and age-related diseases.

Chapter 6: Activating Sirtuins-Lifestyle Choices

Diet and Nutritional Influences on Sirtuin Activity

The connection between diet, nutrition, and the activity of sirtuins is a fascinating area of research, offering insights into how lifestyle choices can impact the aging process and overall health. Sirtuins, known for their roles in cellular function and longevity, are sensitive to the body's metabolic state, which is greatly influenced by diet. This essay explores the dietary and nutritional factors that can modulate sirtuin activity, highlighting the potential of diet as a tool for influencing these key proteins and, by extension, health and aging.

Caloric Restriction and Sirtuin Activation

Caloric restriction (CR), the reduction of calorie intake without malnutrition, is one of the most well-studied dietary interventions known to extend lifespan in various organisms. Research has shown that CR increases the activity of several sirtuins, particularly SIRT1. The mechanism behind this effect involves the increased levels of NAD+, a cofactor required for sirtuin activity. By reducing calorie intake, cells enter a state of energy conservation, leading to an increase in NAD+ levels and subsequent activation of sirtuins. This activation triggers a series of metabolic and physiological changes that contribute to the beneficial effects of CR on health and longevity.

Nutrients That Mimic Caloric Restriction

Given the challenges of long-term caloric restriction in humans, considerable research has focused on identifying nutrients and compounds that can mimic the effects of CR by activating sirtuins. Resveratrol, a polyphenol found in grapes and red wine, is one of the most studied sirtuin activators. It has been shown to activate SIRT1 and mimic some of the beneficial effects of CR, including improved mitochondrial function and increased lifespan in model organisms. Other compounds such as quercetin, found in apples and onions, and pterostilbene, related to resveratrol and found in blueberries, have also been reported to activate sirtuins and exhibit similar health-promoting effects.

Dietary Patterns and Sirtuin Activation

Beyond individual nutrients, specific dietary patterns have been associated with enhanced sirtuin activity. The Mediterranean diet, rich in fruits, vegetables, nuts, whole grains, and olive oil, has been linked to increased sirtuin activity and improved health outcomes. This diet is high in compounds such as polyphenols and omega-3 fatty acids, which are thought to contribute to sirtuin activation and the diet's overall health benefits. Similarly, diets that are high in fiber and low in processed foods and sugars may also support sirtuin activity by promoting a healthy metabolic state and reducing inflammation.

Amino Acid Restriction and Sirtuins

Restricting certain amino acids, particularly methionine, has been shown to have effects similar to overall caloric restriction in terms of extending lifespan and activating sirtuins. Methionine restriction reduces the levels of certain metabolites that inhibit sirtuin activity, thereby indirectly enhancing sirtuin function. This has led to interest in dietary regimens that moderate the intake of methionine-rich foods, such as certain meats and dairy products, as a strategy for activating sirtuins and promoting healthy aging.

Fasting and Intermittent Fasting

Fasting and intermittent fasting regimes, which involve voluntarily abstaining from food for specific periods, have been shown to influence sirtuin activity. These dietary practices increase NAD+ levels and activate sirtuins, particularly SIRT1. Intermittent fasting, which includes various eating patterns such as time-restricted feeding, has gained popularity as a more manageable alternative to continuous caloric restriction, offering similar benefits in terms of sirtuin activation and health improvements.

Challenges and Considerations

While the impact of diet and nutrition on sirtuin activity offers exciting possibilities for health and longevity, there are challenges and considerations to be noted. The effects of dietary compounds on sirtuins can vary greatly between individuals due to differences in genetics, metabolism, and lifestyle. Furthermore, the long-term safety and effectiveness of sirtuin-activating compounds like resveratrol are still under investigation.

Conclusion

In conclusion, diet and nutrition play a significant role in modulating the activity of sirtuins, offering a potentially powerful tool for influencing health and aging. Dietary interventions such as caloric restriction, specific nutrient intake, and fasting regimes can activate sirtuins and trigger beneficial health effects. As research in this area continues to evolve, it holds promise for developing dietary strategies to enhance healthspan and prevent age-related diseases. Understanding the complex interactions between diet, nutrition, and sirtuin activity is key to harnessing the potential of these proteins for improving human health and longevity.

Exercise and Its Effects on Sirtuins

The intersection of exercise and sirtuin activity presents a captivating dimension in the study of aging and health. Sirtuins, known for their regulatory roles in various cellular processes, have been found to be responsive to physical activity. The effects of exercise on sirtuins provide a window into understanding how lifestyle choices can directly impact the molecular mechanisms underlying health and longevity. This essay explores the relationship between exercise and sirtuins, highlighting how physical activity influences these crucial proteins.

The Impact of Exercise on Sirtuin Activation

Exercise, a well-established promoter of health and longevity, has been shown to influence the activity of several sirtuins, particularly SIRT1 and SIRT3. The mechanism behind this influence is multifaceted, involving changes in energy metabolism, oxidative stress, and mitochondrial function. During physical activity, the energy demand of muscles increases, leading to a rise in the levels of NAD+, the cofactor required for sirtuin activity. This increase in NAD+ levels enhances the activity of sirtuins, which in turn modulate various physiological responses to exercise.

SIRT1: Central Player in Exercise-Induced Adaptations

SIRT1, the most studied sirtuin in the context of exercise, plays a pivotal role in mediating the beneficial effects of physical activity. It regulates metabolic pathways in muscle and other tissues, adapting the body to the increased energy demands of exercise. SIRT1 influences fat and glucose metabolism, enhancing insulin sensitivity and fatty acid oxidation – changes that are beneficial for metabolic health and may combat conditions such as obesity and type 2 diabetes.

Moreover, SIRT1 activation during exercise contributes to the improvement of mitochondrial function and efficiency. SIRT1 modulates the activity of PGC-1α, a master regulator of mitochondrial biogenesis, promoting the formation of new mitochondria in muscle cells. This enhancement of mitochondrial capacity is crucial for endurance and overall muscle health, particularly in the context of aging.

SIRT3: Regulator of Mitochondrial Health in Muscle

SIRT3, predominantly located in mitochondria, is another sirtuin significantly influenced by exercise. It plays a key role in regulating mitochondrial metabolism and protecting cells from oxidative damage. During exercise, SIRT3 activity increases, leading to enhanced mitochondrial antioxidant capacity and energy production. This increase in SIRT3 activity is vital for maintaining muscle function and protecting against age-related decline in muscle health.

Exercise, Sirtuins, and Neuroprotection

Beyond muscle health, exercise has been shown to have neuroprotective effects, in part mediated by sirtuins. Exercise induces the expression of SIRT1 in the brain, which can contribute to enhanced cognitive function and protection against neurodegenerative diseases. SIRT1's role in modulating neuroinflammation and oxidative stress in the brain is a key factor in these neuroprotective effects.

The Role of Exercise in Systemic Effects Mediated by Sirtuins

The influence of exercise on sirtuins extends beyond local effects in muscle and brain tissue. Exercise-induced activation of sirtuins can have systemic effects, impacting organs and tissues throughout the body. For instance, exercise-induced changes in SIRT1 activity can influence lipid and glucose metabolism in the liver, enhance insulin sensitivity, and modulate inflammatory responses, contributing to overall metabolic health.

Potential for Exercise as a Therapeutic Strategy

The relationship between exercise and sirtuins opens up potential avenues for using physical activity as a therapeutic strategy in age-related diseases and metabolic disorders. By activating sirtuins, exercise can mimic some of the beneficial effects of caloric restriction and other lifespan-extending interventions. This makes exercise a potentially powerful, non-pharmacological approach to enhancing healthspan and preventing disease.

Challenges and Future Research

While the benefits of exercise on sirtuin activation are clear, challenges remain in fully understanding this relationship. Individual differences in response to exercise, the optimal type and amount of physical activity needed to modulate sirtuin activity effectively, and the long-term implications of these changes require further investigation.

Conclusion

In conclusion, the effects of exercise on sirtuins highlight the profound impact of physical activity on cellular and molecular processes related to health and aging. By activating sirtuins, exercise triggers a cascade of beneficial effects, from enhanced metabolic function and mitochondrial health to neuroprotection and systemic benefits. This understanding reinforces the importance of exercise as a key lifestyle choice for promoting health and longevity. As research in this area continues to evolve, it offers the promise of developing more targeted and effective strategies for harnessing the power of sirtuins through exercise to improve human health and combat age-related diseases.

Chapter 7: Pharmaceutical Pursuits–Drugs Targeting Sirtuins

Current Sirtuin-Activating Compounds

The exploration of sirtuin-activating compounds represents a significant advance in the field of aging and longevity research. Sirtuins, a family of proteins known for their roles in regulating metabolism, stress resistance, and cellular health, have become targets for pharmacological intervention aimed at enhancing healthspan and treating age-related diseases. This essay examines the current landscape of sirtuin-activating compounds, discussing their mechanisms, potential benefits, and the challenges faced in developing these molecules into effective therapies.

Resveratrol: The Pioneer Sirtuin Activator

Resveratrol, a natural polyphenol found in red wine, grapes, and berries, was one of the first compounds identified to activate sirtuins, particularly SIRT1. It gained widespread attention for its potential anti-aging and health-promoting effects. Resveratrol has been shown to mimic some of the beneficial effects of caloric restriction, such as improving mitochondrial function, enhancing stress resistance, and extending lifespan in various model organisms. Its mechanisms of action involve the activation of SIRT1, which leads to the modulation of pathways associated with aging and metabolic regulation.

SRT1720 and Related Synthetic Compounds

Following the discovery of resveratrol, efforts to develop more potent and specific sirtuin activators led to the synthesis of compounds like SRT1720. These synthetic molecules have been designed to more effectively target sirtuins, particularly SIRT1. SRT1720 and its analogs have shown promise in preclinical studies, exhibiting enhanced metabolic and healthspan benefits compared to resveratrol. These compounds have the potential to treat metabolic disorders such as obesity and diabetes by modulating sirtuin activity and improving metabolic efficiency.

NAD+ Precursors: Boosting Sirtuin Activity Indirectly

Given that sirtuins require NAD+ to function, increasing the availability of this coenzyme is another strategy for activating sirtuins. Compounds such as nicotinamide riboside (NR) and nicotinamide mononucleotide (NMN) are NAD+ precursors that can elevate NAD+ levels in cells and tissues. By boosting NAD+ availability, these precursors can indirectly enhance sirtuin activity, leading to improved cellular health and resilience. NAD+ precursors have shown potential in preclinical studies for improving metabolic health, mitigating age-related decline, and enhancing longevity.

Quercetin and Other Natural Flavonoids

Quercetin, a flavonoid present in many fruits and vegetables, has been identified as a sirtuin activator. Similar to resveratrol, quercetin exerts its effects partly by activating SIRT1. It has shown potential in reducing inflammation, improving endothelial function, and enhancing stress resistance. Other natural flavonoids with similar properties are also being studied for their ability to modulate sirtuin activity and confer health benefits.

Challenges in Developing Sirtuin-Activating Drugs

Despite the promise shown by these compounds, there are significant challenges in developing sirtuin activators as therapeutic agents. One major challenge is ensuring specificity and avoiding off-target effects, which can lead to adverse reactions. Additionally, the long-term effects and safety profiles of these compounds need thorough investigation, especially given the broad impact of sirtuins on cellular function.

The bioavailability and effective dosage of natural compounds like resveratrol and quercetin in humans also pose challenges. While these compounds show beneficial effects in laboratory settings, achieving effective concentrations in human tissues can be difficult without high doses, which may not be practical or safe.

Furthermore, the complexity of aging as a biological process means that modulating sirtuins alone may not be sufficient to address all aspects of aging and age-related diseases. A comprehensive approach, possibly involving a combination of lifestyle interventions and pharmacological treatments, might be necessary for maximal benefit.

Future Directions and Potential

The field of sirtuin-activating compounds is evolving, with ongoing research aimed at improving the efficacy, specificity, and safety of these molecules. Advances in drug design and delivery methods may overcome current limitations, leading to more effective therapies.

In conclusion, the development of sirtuin-activating compounds represents an exciting area of research with significant potential for improving health and treating age-related diseases. These compounds, ranging from natural polyphenols to synthetic molecules and NAD+ precursors, offer various strategies for modulating sirtuin activity. While challenges remain in translating these findings into effective therapies, the progress in this field holds promise for future interventions aimed at enhancing longevity and mitigating the impact of aging.

Clinical Trials and Challenges in Drug Development

The journey from discovering potential therapeutic compounds to their successful implementation as drugs involves a complex and rigorous process, encompassing clinical trials and numerous developmental challenges. When it comes to drugs targeting sirtuins, a group of proteins implicated in aging and metabolic regulation, this journey is fraught with unique hurdles and considerations. This essay delves into the landscape of clinical trials for sirtuin-targeting drugs and the myriad challenges encountered in their development, emphasizing the intricate path from laboratory research to clinical application.

The Landscape of Clinical Trials for Sirtuin-Targeting Drugs

Clinical trials for sirtuin-targeting drugs have primarily focused on compounds like resveratrol, SRT1720, and NAD+ precursors such as nicotinamide riboside. These trials aim to validate the efficacy and safety of these compounds in treating age-related diseases or improving healthspan. For instance, resveratrol has been studied in numerous clinical trials for its potential benefits in cardiovascular health, diabetes, and neurodegenerative diseases. Similarly, trials involving NAD+ precursors have examined their impact on metabolic health, mitochondrial function, and aging biomarkers.

Challenges in Efficacy and Specificity

One of the key challenges in developing sirtuin-targeting drugs is ensuring their efficacy. Many compounds that show promising results in cellular and animal models do not always translate into effective treatments in humans. This discrepancy can be due to differences in metabolism, bioavailability, and the complexity of human physiology compared to laboratory models.

Another major issue is the specificity of these compounds. Sirtuins are a family of proteins with multiple members, each having distinct and sometimes overlapping functions. Designing drugs that specifically target one sirtuin without affecting others is challenging. Off-target effects can lead to unintended consequences, complicating the drug development process.

Addressing Safety and Long-Term Effects

Safety is a paramount concern in drug development, especially for compounds meant to be used over long periods, as would be the case for anti-aging drugs. Assessing the long-term safety of sirtuin-activating compounds is crucial, given the broad role of these proteins in cellular function. Potential side effects, interactions with other medications, and impacts on various physiological systems must be thoroughly evaluated.

The Complexities of Aging as a Target

Targeting aging itself presents a unique set of challenges. Aging is a multifactorial process with numerous contributing factors, including genetics, lifestyle, and environmental influences. A drug that targets one aspect of aging, such as sirtuin activity, may not address other critical factors contributing to age-related decline. Moreover, measuring the effectiveness of anti-aging drugs requires long-term studies and reliable biomarkers of aging, which are currently limited.

Regulatory Hurdles and Approval Processes

The regulatory approval process for new drugs is stringent and often lengthy, posing another layer of challenge. Anti-aging drugs must demonstrate clear benefits in preventing, delaying, or reversing age-related conditions, which can be difficult to quantify. Furthermore, regulatory agencies like the FDA have specific criteria for drug approval, which may not fully align with the goals of anti-aging therapeutics.

Variability in Human Populations

Human populations are genetically and environmentally diverse, leading to variability in responses to sirtuin-targeting drugs. Personalized medicine approaches may be necessary to optimize the benefits of these treatments for individual patients. This requires a deeper understanding of genetic and lifestyle factors that influence individual responses to these drugs.

Financial and Ethical Considerations

Drug development is an expensive endeavor, and the cost can be particularly high for pioneering treatments like sirtuin-targeting drugs. Securing funding and navigating the cost-benefit landscape is a significant challenge. Ethical considerations also come into play, particularly in the context of anti-aging treatments. Issues of access, equity, and the societal implications of extending human lifespan must be considered.

Future Directions and Potential

Despite these challenges, the potential of sirtuin-targeting drugs remains significant. Ongoing research and advancements in drug design, personalized medicine, and aging biomarkers continue to drive the field forward. Collaborative efforts between researchers, clinicians, and regulatory bodies are crucial in overcoming these hurdles and realizing the potential of these innovative therapies.

Conclusion

In conclusion, the path to developing effective sirtuin-targeting drugs is laden with challenges, from ensuring efficacy and safety to navigating complex regulatory and ethical landscapes. Clinical trials play a crucial role in this journey, serving as the bridge between laboratory discoveries and clinical applications. As the field of sirtuin research advances, it offers the promise of groundbreaking treatments that could profoundly impact how we approach aging and age-related diseases. The journey, though fraught with obstacles, is a testament to the relentless pursuit of medical science to improve human health and longevity. The success of this endeavor will not only depend on scientific and technological advancements but also on a holistic approach that considers the ethical, social, and economic dimensions of extending human lifespans. As we continue to explore the frontiers of aging and sirtuin biology, the potential for transformative therapies looms on the horizon, heralding a new era in medicine where aging might be treated not as an inevitable decline, but as a modifiable aspect of human biology. The road ahead is complex, but the rewards – a healthier, longer life for future generations – make this journey one of the most exciting and significant in the realm of modern scientific research.

Chapter 8: Ethics and Implications of Prolonging Human Life

Ethical Considerations in Longevity Research

The field of longevity research, particularly as it edges closer to tangible results in extending human life, brings to light numerous ethical considerations. These considerations are not just confined to the realms of medical ethics but extend to broader societal and philosophical realms. This essay explores the multifaceted ethical issues surrounding longevity research, highlighting the need for a balanced and thoughtful approach as we advance in our understanding and capabilities of extending human life.

The Quest for Longevity: Balancing Benefits and Risks

The primary goal of longevity research is to extend the human lifespan, ideally coupled with an extended healthspan. While the benefits of such advancements are clear, including reduced suffering from age-related diseases and enhanced quality of life in later years, there are inherent risks and ethical dilemmas. One major concern is the unintended consequences of significantly altering the human lifespan. Extending life may bring unforeseen medical, psychological, and social challenges that we are yet ill-equipped to handle. The ethicality of pursuing such research hinges on a careful analysis of these benefits and risks.

Equity and Access to Longevity Interventions

A critical ethical issue in longevity research is the question of access and equity. There is a potential risk that life-extending treatments might only be available to the wealthy or those in developed countries, exacerbating existing health and social inequalities. Ensuring equitable access to the benefits of longevity research is paramount to avoid a scenario where lifespan becomes yet another commodity that widens the gap between different socioeconomic groups.

The Impact on Population Dynamics and Resource Allocation

Significantly extending human lifespans will have profound implications for population dynamics. Concerns include overpopulation, resource depletion, and environmental impacts. Ethical longevity research must consider these factors, ensuring that advances in extending life do not compromise the wellbeing of the planet and future generations. Furthermore, there are implications for healthcare systems, pension schemes, and the workforce, which will all need to adapt to a population with a substantially extended lifespan.

Autonomy and the Individual's Right to Choose

Respecting individual autonomy is a key principle in medical ethics. In the context of longevity research, this translates to the right of individuals to choose whether or not to pursue treatments that extend life. The ethical framework of longevity research must ensure that individuals are fully informed and able to make autonomous decisions about undergoing such interventions.

The Naturalness Argument and the Role of Medicine

A philosophical debate in the ethics of longevity research revolves around the concept of naturalness. Some argue that extending human life beyond its current biological limits is unnatural and goes against the natural course of life. However, others contend that medicine has always sought to extend life and improve health, making longevity research a natural progression of medical science. Navigating this debate requires a nuanced understanding of the role of medicine and the goals of healthcare.

Societal and Cultural Implications

Longevity research has far-reaching societal and cultural implications. Culturally, how we perceive aging and the value we place on different stages of life may shift significantly. Societally, extended lifespans could lead to changes in how we structure education, career development, retirement, and intergenerational relationships. Ethical considerations must include these broader cultural and societal impacts.

Psychological Well-being and Quality of Life

Extending lifespan raises questions about the quality of life in the additional years. Ethical longevity research must focus not only on quantity of life but also on the quality, ensuring that extended life is coupled with health, well-being, and fulfillment. Psychological impacts, such as the potential for extended grief or changes in life planning and aspirations, must also be considered.

The Burden of Prolonged Aging

Another ethical concern is the potential burden of prolonged aging. If the extension of life does not equally extend healthspan, there could be an increase in the population suffering from the ailments and dependencies of old age. The ethical approach to longevity research should prioritize interventions that enhance healthspan, not just lifespan.

Conclusion

In conclusion, the ethical considerations in longevity research are diverse and complex, encompassing medical, societal, philosophical, and psychological dimensions. As we advance in our scientific understanding and capabilities to extend human life, it is imperative that these ethical considerations are at the forefront of research and policy discussions. Balancing the pursuit of extended life with careful consideration of the implications for individuals, society, and the planet is essential. Ethical longevity research should aim not just for longer life, but for a life that is meaningful, equitable, and sustainable for all.

Social and Economic Impacts of Extended Lifespans

The prospect of significantly extending human lifespans through advancements in science, particularly in fields like sirtuin research, raises profound social and economic questions. While the idea of living longer, healthier lives is appealing, it also brings to the fore a plethora of implications that society must grapple with. This essay examines the multifaceted social and economic impacts of extended lifespans, exploring how such a fundamental shift could reshape demographics, healthcare, the economy, and ethical frameworks.

Demographic Changes and Challenges

One of the most immediate impacts of extended lifespans would be on the demographic structure of societies. A significant increase in life expectancy could lead to an aging population on an unprecedented scale. While an older population can bring a wealth of experience and wisdom, it also raises concerns about age-related dependency ratios. There would be more people requiring care and support for a longer duration, potentially straining social support systems and caregiving resources.

Healthcare Systems Under Pressure

Extended lifespans would inevitably place additional demands on healthcare systems. With more people living longer, the prevalence of age-related diseases, even if delayed, could increase, requiring more extensive healthcare resources. This situation would necessitate a reevaluation of healthcare infrastructure, including long-term care facilities, healthcare financing, and medical workforce training. The focus might also shift more towards preventive care and managing chronic conditions effectively over a longer period.

Economic Implications: Workforce and Retirement

The traditional models of employment and retirement would be challenged by longer lifespans. With more years of life, the working age could be extended, potentially altering career trajectories and concepts of retirement. This shift could have benefits, such as increased experience and knowledge in the workforce, but also challenges, including potential ageism and the need for continuous skill development in an ever-evolving job market.

From an economic perspective, extended working years could contribute positively to national economies by maintaining a larger, more experienced workforce. However, it also raises questions about job opportunities for younger generations and the need for intergenerational equity in job markets.

Social Dynamics and Intergenerational Relationships

Longer lifespans would also impact social dynamics, particularly intergenerational relationships. Family structures could evolve, with more generations coexisting simultaneously. This could lead to strengthened intergenerational bonds but also potential conflicts and pressures, as resources and responsibilities are negotiated across extended families.

Impact on Pensions and Social Security

The financial models underpinning pensions and social security systems are based on current life expectancy trends. A significant increase in lifespan would strain these systems, requiring rethinking and restructuring to ensure sustainability. Governments and policymakers would need to consider how to fund these programs in the face of extended retirement periods.

Ethical Considerations and Equality

The possibility of extended lifespans raises profound ethical questions, particularly concerning equality and access. If life-extending technologies and treatments are expensive, they could widen the existing health and socioeconomic disparities. Ensuring equitable access to these advancements becomes a moral imperative, necessitating global cooperation and policy frameworks that prioritize fairness and inclusivity.

Psychological and Cultural Impacts

Living significantly longer lives would also have psychological and cultural impacts. Societies would need to adjust their attitudes towards aging and the life course. Individuals might approach life planning, education, and personal development differently, knowing they have more time. This could lead to a cultural shift in how life stages are perceived and experienced.

Environmental Considerations

Longer lifespans also bring environmental considerations. More people living longer could result in increased consumption and strain on environmental resources. Sustainable living and environmental conservation would become even more critical to ensure that the planet can support a larger, longer-living population.

Conclusion

In conclusion, the social and economic impacts of extended lifespans are vast and complex, touching upon every aspect of society. While the potential benefits of longer, healthier lives are immense, they come with challenges that require careful, proactive planning and policy-making. Addressing these issues effectively will require a multidisciplinary approach, combining insights from science, economics, ethics, and social sciences. As we stand on the cusp of potentially life-extending scientific breakthroughs, it is imperative to consider and prepare for the broader implications they bring to ensure that the benefits are shared equitably and sustainably across society.

Chapter 9: Personalized Approaches to Longevity

Sirtuins and Personalized Medicine

The integration of sirtuin research into the field of personalized medicine represents a groundbreaking stride in our quest to understand and influence the aging process. Personalized medicine, with its focus on individual variability in genes, environment, and lifestyle, is particularly relevant when considering interventions targeting sirtuins, a family of proteins intricately involved in various aspects of aging and cellular regulation. This essay explores the potential role of sirtuins in personalized medicine, particularly in the context of longevity and age-related diseases, and the challenges and opportunities that lie ahead in this promising field.

The Role of Sirtuins in Cellular Function

Sirtuins, known primarily for their roles in aging, also play a significant part in metabolic regulation, DNA repair, and stress resistance. They are a point of convergence for numerous cellular pathways, responding to environmental signals such as nutrient availability and stress factors. This makes them a prime target for interventions aiming to modulate aging and associated pathologies. The diverse functions of sirtuins across different cell types and tissues add a layer of complexity, which personalized medicine aims to unravel.

Personalized Medicine: Tailoring Sirtuin-Targeted Interventions

Personalized medicine seeks to tailor medical treatment to the individual characteristics of each patient. In the context of sirtuins, this approach involves understanding how individual differences in genetic makeup, lifestyle, and environmental factors influence sirtuin activity and the aging process. For example, variations in genes encoding sirtuins or enzymes involved in their regulation might affect how individuals respond to certain diets, drugs, or lifestyle interventions targeting sirtuin pathways.

Genetic Variability and Sirtuin Function

Genetic variability plays a crucial role in the functioning of sirtuins. Polymorphisms in sirtuin genes can lead to differences in their expression or activity, influencing susceptibility to aging and various diseases. Personalized medicine aims to identify these genetic variations and understand their implications for health and longevity. This knowledge can then be used to develop targeted interventions, such as specific dietary recommendations or pharmacological agents, to modulate sirtuin activity effectively.

Lifestyle Factors, Diet, and Sirtuin Modulation

The activity of sirtuins is highly responsive to lifestyle factors, particularly diet and physical activity. Nutrients that affect cellular energy levels, such as glucose and fatty acids, can influence sirtuin activity. Personalized nutrition, which considers individual dietary habits, metabolic status, and genetic background, can be a powerful approach to modulate sirtuin activity for optimal health and longevity. Similarly, personalized exercise programs tailored to an individual's fitness level, health status, and genetic predispositions can optimize sirtuin activation.

Pharmacogenomics and Sirtuin-Targeting Drugs

Pharmacogenomics, the study of how genes affect a person's response to drugs, is a critical component of personalized medicine. Sirtuin-targeting drugs, such as sirtuin activators or inhibitors, can have varying effects based on an individual's genetic makeup. Understanding these genetic differences can help in selecting the most appropriate and effective sirtuin-targeted therapies for each individual, minimizing adverse effects and maximizing therapeutic benefits.

Biomarkers of Aging and Sirtuin Activity

Developing reliable biomarkers of aging is a key objective in personalized medicine. Sirtuins themselves, or the molecular pathways they influence, could serve as potential biomarkers. Monitoring these biomarkers can provide insights into an individual's biological aging process, allowing for early intervention and monitoring of the effectiveness of sirtuin-targeted therapies.

Challenges and Ethical Considerations

The application of sirtuins in personalized medicine is not without challenges. The complexity of sirtuin pathways, their interactions with other cellular processes, and the influence of a myriad of external factors make it difficult to predict individual responses to interventions accurately. Additionally, ethical considerations, including privacy concerns related to genetic information and equitable access to personalized therapies, must be addressed.

Future Prospects

The future of sirtuins in personalized medicine holds great promise. Advances in genomics, bioinformatics, and a deeper understanding of sirtuin biology could lead to more precise and effective interventions for aging and age-related diseases. The potential to not only extend lifespan but also enhance healthspan could have profound implications for how we age and how we approach the treatment of aging-related conditions.

Conclusion

In conclusion, the intersection of sirtuin research and personalized medicine offers exciting prospects for the future of healthcare and longevity. By tailoring interventions to individual genetic, environmental, and lifestyle factors, we can optimize the role of sirtuins in promoting health and longevity. The path forward involves a multidisciplinary approach, combining insights from genetics, molecular biology, nutrition, pharmacology, and ethics. As we continue to unravel the complexities of sirtuins and their interactions with our unique biological makeup, the potential to personalize our approach to aging and disease grows ever closer, promising a future where longevity is not only about adding years to life but also life to years.

Genetic Testing and Individualized Lifestyle Interventions

In the realm of personalized medicine, genetic testing and individualized lifestyle interventions have emerged as key components in the pursuit of longevity and enhanced healthspan. This approach is grounded in the understanding that genetic makeup can significantly influence how individuals respond to various lifestyle factors, such as diet, exercise, and environmental stressors. By tailoring lifestyle interventions based on genetic information, it is possible to optimize health outcomes and potentially slow the aging process. This essay explores the interplay between genetic testing and individualized lifestyle interventions, highlighting their potential in personalizing approaches to longevity.

The Role of Genetic Testing in Personalized Medicine

Genetic testing has revolutionized the field of personalized medicine by providing insights into individual susceptibilities to diseases, responses to specific nutrients, and potential reactions to physical activities. With advances in genomics, it is now possible to identify genetic variants that affect the metabolism of vitamins, the efficacy of certain exercises, and the risk of developing age-related diseases. This genetic information can be instrumental in designing personalized lifestyle interventions that cater to the unique needs of each individual.

Personalized Nutrition: Tailoring Diets to Genetic Profiles

One of the most significant applications of genetic testing in personalized medicine is in the field of nutrition. Genetic variations can influence nutrient absorption, metabolism, and even food preferences. For instance, variations in genes related to lipid metabolism can dictate how an individual processes fats, impacting their risk for cardiovascular diseases. Similarly, genetic differences in vitamin D receptors can affect the efficiency of vitamin D metabolism. By understanding these genetic predispositions, nutritionists can develop tailored dietary plans that enhance nutrient uptake and minimize the risk of diet-related diseases.

Exercise and Physical Activity: A Genetic Perspective

Physical exercise, a cornerstone of healthy aging, can also be optimized through genetic testing. Genetic variations can affect muscle composition, endurance, and recovery rates after exercise. Some individuals may benefit more from endurance activities, while others may see better results from strength training. Genetic testing can guide the development of personalized exercise programs that maximize health benefits and reduce the risk of injuries, making physical activity more effective and enjoyable.

Stress Management and Environmental Interactions

Genetic testing can also shed light on how individuals respond to stress and environmental factors. Genetic predispositions can influence the psychological and physiological responses to stress, which is a known factor in aging and health. By understanding these genetic factors, personalized strategies for stress management, such as mindfulness practices, yoga, or other relaxation techniques, can be implemented more effectively.

The Role of Epigenetics in Aging and Lifestyle Interventions

Epigenetics, the study of changes in gene expression that do not involve alterations to the underlying DNA sequence, is another important aspect of personalized medicine. Lifestyle factors such as diet, exercise, and stress can cause epigenetic modifications that influence aging and disease processes. Understanding individual epigenetic profiles can provide further insights into the most effective lifestyle interventions for promoting longevity.

Challenges and Considerations in Implementing Personalized Interventions

While the potential of genetic testing and personalized interventions is vast, there are several challenges and considerations in their implementation. The accuracy and interpretation of genetic tests are crucial, as the field of genomics is still evolving. Moreover, the integration of genetic information into practical lifestyle recommendations requires a multidisciplinary approach involving geneticists, nutritionists, exercise physiologists, and other healthcare professionals.

Ethical, Privacy, and Equity Issues

Ethical and privacy concerns are paramount in the field of genetic testing. The handling of sensitive genetic data must be done with utmost care to protect individual privacy. Additionally, there is a need to address equity issues, ensuring that the benefits of personalized medicine are accessible to all segments of the population, regardless of socioeconomic status.

Future Perspectives

The future of personalized medicine, particularly in the context of longevity, looks promising. As research continues to uncover the complex interactions between genetics, lifestyle, and aging, the potential for tailored interventions to enhance healthspan becomes increasingly attainable. The integration of genetic testing with comprehensive lifestyle interventions could usher in a new era of preventive medicine, where the focus shifts from treating disease to maintaining health and vitality throughout life.

Conclusion

In conclusion, the synergy between genetic testing and individualized lifestyle interventions holds immense potential in the pursuit of longevity and optimal health. By understanding the unique genetic makeup of individuals, it is possible to tailor lifestyle interventions to maximize their efficacy and minimize risks. As we advance in our understanding of genetics, lifestyle, and their impact on aging, personalized approaches to health and longevity will likely become an integral part of healthcare, offering a more proactive and preventive strategy to maintaining wellness throughout the lifespan.

Chapter 10:
The Future of Ageless Living

Emerging Research and Potential Discoveries

The realm of ageless living is rapidly advancing, fueled by emerging research and potential discoveries that promise to reshape our understanding of aging and longevity. This field stands at the forefront of biomedical science, where innovative studies and technological breakthroughs converge to unveil new pathways for enhancing healthspan and potentially altering the human aging process. This essay explores the current landscape of emerging research in ageless living, highlighting the potential discoveries that could revolutionize our approach to aging and longevity.

Advancements in Cellular and Molecular Understanding of Aging

One of the most exciting areas of research in ageless living is the deepening understanding of the cellular and molecular mechanisms of aging. Groundbreaking studies are unraveling the complex interplay between genetics, metabolism, and environmental factors that contribute to aging. Key areas of focus include telomere biology, mitochondrial function, stem cell rejuvenation, and the role of cellular senescence in age-related decline. Discoveries in these areas could lead to novel interventions that target the fundamental causes of aging, rather than merely treating its symptoms.

Sirtuins and Longevity Pathways

The research into sirtuins and related longevity pathways continues to be a hotbed of potential discoveries. Sirtuins, known for their role in extending lifespan in various organisms, are being studied for their broader implications in human aging. Advances in understanding how sirtuins regulate cellular processes like DNA repair, metabolism, and stress responses could pave the way for new treatments that enhance longevity and mitigate age-related diseases.

The Promise of Regenerative Medicine

Regenerative medicine holds immense potential in the quest for ageless living. This field focuses on repairing, replacing, or regenerating human cells, tissues, or organs to restore or establish normal function. Breakthroughs in stem cell therapy, tissue engineering, and organ regeneration could lead to revolutionary treatments for age-related conditions and injuries, offering the potential to rejuvenate aging tissues and organs.

Nutrigenomics and Personalized Nutrition

Nutrigenomics, the study of the interaction between nutrition and genes, is gaining traction as a critical component of ageless living. This field explores how individual genetic variations affect responses to nutrients and dietary patterns, influencing aging and health outcomes. Personalized nutrition, tailored to individual genetic profiles, could optimize dietary interventions to slow aging and prevent age-related diseases.

AI and Big Data in Aging Research

Artificial intelligence (AI) and big data are becoming increasingly important in aging research. AI algorithms can analyze vast amounts of genetic, metabolic, and clinical data to identify patterns and predict individual responses to treatments. This technology could accelerate the discovery of anti-aging compounds, improve the personalization of healthcare, and uncover novel insights into the aging process.

The Microbiome and Aging

The human microbiome, the community of microorganisms living in and on our bodies, is emerging as a key factor in aging and longevity. Research is revealing how changes in the microbiome composition can influence aging, immune function, and susceptibility to age-related diseases. Modulating the microbiome through diet, probiotics, or other interventions could become a vital strategy in promoting healthy aging.

Lifestyle Interventions and Behavioral Science

Lifestyle interventions, including diet, exercise, and stress management, remain central to ageless living. Emerging research in behavioral science is focusing on how to effectively implement and sustain these lifestyle changes. Understanding the psychological and social factors that influence aging-related behaviors could enhance the effectiveness of lifestyle interventions in promoting longevity.

Ethical, Social, and Policy Implications

As research in ageless living progresses, it raises important ethical, social, and policy questions. Issues such as equitable access to anti-aging interventions, the societal implications of extended lifespans, and the ethical considerations of manipulating the human lifespan are becoming increasingly relevant. Addressing these issues is crucial for the responsible advancement of ageless living research.

Conclusion

In conclusion, the future of ageless living is brimming with potential, driven by a confluence of emerging research across various scientific disciplines. From molecular breakthroughs to advances in regenerative medicine, nutrigenomics, and AI, the field is poised for significant discoveries that could profoundly impact our understanding and management of aging. As we navigate this exciting frontier, a holistic approach that considers the ethical, social, and policy aspects of extending human healthspan will be essential.

The journey towards ageless living is not just a scientific endeavor but a collective quest that holds the promise of transforming our experience of aging and opening new possibilities for health and vitality in the later stages of life.

Philosophical Perspectives on Eternal Youth

The quest for eternal youth, a theme as old as human civilization itself, has always been intertwined with philosophical inquiry. In contemporary times, as scientific advancements bring the prospect of significantly prolonged youthfulness closer to reality, it becomes imperative to explore the philosophical implications of this pursuit. This essay delves into the philosophical perspectives surrounding eternal youth, examining the ethical, existential, and societal dimensions that such a paradigm shift in human lifespan and healthspan would entail.

The Ethical Dimension of Eternal Youth

At the heart of the philosophical discourse on eternal youth is the question of ethics. Extending youthfulness indefinitely or significantly poses ethical challenges that society must grapple with. One of the primary concerns is the issue of access and equity. If treatments or technologies enabling prolonged youth are expensive or scarce, they could widen existing social inequalities, with longer, healthier lives becoming a privilege of the affluent. This raises fundamental questions about justice and fairness in society.

Moreover, the ethics of altering a natural process such as aging is a contentious issue. Some argue that striving for eternal youth is a manifestation of human hubris, an attempt to transcend natural limitations, while others see it as a continuation of the human quest to overcome biological constraints and improve the quality of life.

Existential and Psychological Implications

The prospect of eternal youth also brings existential questions to the fore. Aging and the awareness of mortality are deeply embedded in the human experience, influencing our values, aspirations, and understanding of life. Prolonged youth could fundamentally alter our perception of life stages, achievements, and the passage of time.

There are concerns about the psychological impact of extended youthfulness. Would the extension of youth lead to a perpetual adolescence, with individuals taking longer to mature and accept responsibilities? Or would it result in richer, more varied life experiences, with individuals having more time to explore different facets of life?

The Impact on Identity and Personal Development

The concept of identity is closely linked to the passage of time and life experiences. Prolonging youth raises questions about personal development and identity formation. Traditionally, aging is associated with gaining wisdom and experience. If this process is significantly altered, how would it impact individual and collective wisdom? Would the extended time in a youthful state facilitate continuous growth and learning, or would it lead to stagnation?

Societal and Cultural Shifts

Eternal youth would inevitably lead to significant shifts in societal and cultural norms. Traditionally, societies are structured around life stages, with expectations and roles changing as individuals age. Prolonged youthfulness would require a rethinking of these structures, including education, career development, and retirement. Culturally, the perception of aging, which is often viewed negatively, could undergo a transformation, potentially leading to a more age-inclusive society.

The Value of Aging and Mortality

Philosophically, aging and mortality are often seen as essential aspects of the human condition, imparting urgency and meaning to life. The quest for eternal youth challenges this view, prompting a reevaluation of the value we place on aging. Is the natural aging process something to be combatted, or does it have intrinsic value that contributes to the richness of the human experience?

Balancing Individual Desires and Collective Good

The pursuit of eternal youth also raises questions about the balance between individual desires and the collective good. While the desire for prolonged youthfulness is understandable at an individual level, its implications at a societal and environmental level are complex. Overpopulation, resource allocation, and environmental sustainability are just a few of the issues that need consideration.

Technological Hubris and Human Nature

Finally, the philosophical debate on eternal youth touches on the theme of technological hubris and the limits of human nature. The relentless pursuit of technological solutions to biological problems, such as aging, reflects a broader narrative about humanity's relationship with nature and technology. It prompts us to consider the boundaries of human intervention in natural processes and the consequences of crossing these boundaries.

Conclusion

In conclusion, the philosophical perspectives on eternal youth are as diverse as they are profound. The ethical, existential, and societal implications of significantly prolonging youthfulness extend beyond the realm of science into the core of human values and existence. As scientific advancements make the prospect of extended youth a real possibility, it becomes increasingly important to engage in these philosophical discourses, ensuring that the path forward is navigated with wisdom, foresight, and a deep understanding of the intricate tapestry of the human condition. The pursuit of eternal youth, while offering exciting possibilities, must be approached with a balanced perspective that considers not only the potential benefits but also the profound and far-reaching implications for individuals and society at large.

Chapter 11: Conclusion–The Reality of Seeking Eternal Youth

Summarizing the Potential and Limits of Sirtuin Research

In the quest to understand and potentially extend human life, sirtuin research has emerged as a beacon of hope, offering insights into the molecular mechanisms of aging and longevity. Sirtuins, a family of proteins involved in various cellular processes, have been at the center of significant scientific inquiry and debate. This essay aims to encapsulate the potential and limitations of sirtuin research, providing a balanced perspective on what we can realistically expect from this exciting field of study.

The Potential of Sirtuin Research

Advancing Understanding of Aging

One of the most significant contributions of sirtuin research has been the deepening understanding of the biological processes of aging. Sirtuins have been found to play critical roles in DNA repair, metabolic regulation, stress resistance, and inflammation, all of which are central to the aging process. This knowledge has been instrumental in identifying potential targets for anti-aging interventions.

Potential for Disease Prevention and Treatment

Sirtuins are implicated in numerous age-related diseases, including neurodegenerative disorders, cardiovascular diseases, and metabolic syndromes. The modulation of sirtuin activity presents promising avenues for the prevention and treatment of these conditions. By targeting the underlying mechanisms of these diseases, sirtuin-based therapies could offer more effective and holistic treatments compared to those addressing symptoms alone.

Insights into Caloric Restriction and Lifestyle Interventions

Research on sirtuins has also shed light on the mechanisms behind the beneficial effects of caloric restriction on lifespan. Understanding how lifestyle factors such as diet and exercise influence sirtuin activity could lead to the development of interventions that mimic these effects, offering practical ways to enhance health and longevity.

The Limitations of Sirtuin Research

Complexity of Aging

Despite the advancements in sirtuin research, aging remains an incredibly complex process influenced by a myriad of genetic, environmental, and lifestyle factors. Sirtuins are but one piece of this intricate puzzle. The notion that manipulating a single family of proteins could drastically alter the human lifespan is an oversimplification of the aging process.

Challenges in Translating Research to Therapies

Translating findings from sirtuin research into effective therapies has proven challenging. Many compounds that show promise in activating sirtuins or mimicking their effects in cell cultures and animal models have not yielded consistent results in human clinical trials. The discrepancy underscores the challenges in translating laboratory research into viable clinical treatments.

Potential Side Effects and Unintended Consequences

The modulation of sirtuin activity could have unforeseen side effects, given the widespread involvement of these proteins in various cellular functions. Long-term impacts of altering sirtuin pathways are still not fully understood. Caution is necessary to ensure that the pursuit of longevity does not inadvertently lead to adverse health outcomes.

Ethical and Societal Implications

The prospect of significantly extending human lifespan raises profound ethical and societal questions. Issues of access and equity, the impact on population dynamics and resource allocation, and the psychological and societal implications of extended lifespans need careful consideration.

Balancing Expectations with Reality

While sirtuin research holds tremendous promise, it is essential to balance optimism with a realistic understanding of the current state of knowledge. The field is still evolving, with many unanswered questions and challenges to overcome. It is unlikely that sirtuin research alone will unlock the secret to eternal youth or drastically extend human lifespan in the near future.

Future Prospects

Looking ahead, the future of sirtuin research lies in a more integrated approach, combining insights from genetics, molecular biology, and lifestyle studies. Collaboration across various disciplines will be essential in unraveling the complexities of aging and developing effective interventions.

Conclusion

In conclusion, sirtuin research stands as a critical area in the study of aging, offering valuable insights and potential pathways for enhancing human health and longevity. However, it is important to approach this field with a clear understanding of its potential and limitations. As we continue to explore the mysteries of aging, sirtuin research will undoubtedly contribute to this journey, but it is not the panacea for achieving eternal youth. The real value of this research lies in its contribution to a broader, more nuanced understanding of aging, paving the way for interventions that enhance the quality of life, rather than merely extending its duration.

The Balance of Scientific Advancement and Natural Aging

In the modern era, where scientific advancements continually push the boundaries of what is possible, the pursuit of eternal youth stands at a fascinating intersection. This quest, deeply rooted in human history and mythology, is no longer confined to the realms of fantasy but is increasingly entering the realm of scientific plausibility. However, this pursuit raises profound questions about the balance between embracing scientific advancements and respecting the natural process of aging. This essay explores the delicate equilibrium between the desire to extend youth through scientific means and the acceptance of aging as an inherent part of the human experience.

The Allure of Scientific Breakthroughs

The appeal of defying age and prolonging youth is undeniable in a society that often equates youth with beauty, vitality, and productivity. Scientific advancements, particularly in fields like genetics, biotechnology, and medicine, have made significant strides in understanding and potentially manipulating the biological processes of aging. From the discovery of telomerase to the study of sirtuins and the development of regenerative medicine, each breakthrough brings with it the promise of extending healthy human life.

Aging: A Natural and Complex Process

Despite these advancements, aging remains a complex and multifaceted process that is only partially understood. It is a natural part of life, intricately woven into the fabric of human existence. Aging is not merely a biological phenomenon but also a psychological and social one, contributing to the depth and richness of human experience. The acceptance of aging, with its accompanying changes and eventualities, is a part of what makes the human journey profound and meaningful.

Ethical Considerations in the Quest for Youth

The pursuit of eternal youth through scientific means is fraught with ethical considerations. One of the primary concerns is the potential for exacerbating social inequalities. Access to life-extending technologies could be limited to those with financial means, leading to a society where longevity is a commodity available only to the wealthy. Additionally, there are moral questions about the long-term implications of significantly extending human lifespan, including overpopulation and the environmental impact of sustaining a larger, longer-living population.

Psychological Impacts and Societal Shifts

Extending youthfulness could also have profound psychological and societal impacts. It could alter traditional life stages, affect how individuals plan and live their lives, and change societal perceptions of aging and the elderly. There is the potential for both positive and negative consequences, from extended periods of productivity and creativity to challenges in adapting to a new social paradigm where old age is significantly delayed or altered.

Balancing Advancement with Respect for Nature

Finding a balance between harnessing scientific advancements to improve human health and respecting the natural process of aging is crucial. While science offers the potential to prevent or alleviate the ailments associated with aging, there is a need to approach this endeavor with humility and caution. Respecting the natural cycle of life and death, while striving to enhance the quality of life, is a delicate but necessary balance.

The Role of Personal Choice and Diversity

Individual perspectives on aging and the desire for prolonged youth vary widely. Personal choice plays a significant role in how one approaches aging and the use of science to influence this process. Respecting this diversity of views is essential in a society where scientific options for extending youth may become increasingly available.

Preparing for a Future with Extended Youth

As science continues to advance the possibility of extended youthfulness, it is essential to prepare for the societal, ethical, and psychological implications. This preparation involves not only advancing medical and scientific research but also engaging in broad societal dialogues, developing equitable policies, and fostering a culture that values aging as well as youth.

Conclusion

In conclusion, the balance between scientific advancement and natural aging is a complex and evolving narrative. As we stand on the brink of significant breakthroughs in prolonging youth and potentially altering the human aging process, it is crucial to navigate this path with careful consideration of the ethical, societal, and psychological implications. The quest for eternal youth, while holding promise for improved health and vitality, must be tempered with respect for the natural aging process and an understanding of the richness it brings to human life. Balancing these two aspects – the desire for extended youth and the acceptance of aging – will be one of the defining challenges of our time as we forge ahead into an era where the boundaries of human life are continually redefined.